Cell phone radiation and damage

Ramón Martínez López

ISBN: 9798651555093

Contents

Cell phone radiation and damage

INTRODUCTION

Now we are witnessing the arrival of 5G or at least 4G +. The safety of this exposure has never been demonstrated. On the contrary, evidence of its harmfulness is accumulating. In addition, since 2011, the RF / MO electromagnetic radiation from wireless technologies has been considered by the WHO to be possibly carcinogenic (class 2B), largely due to the increased risks of gliomas and acoustic neuromas among long-term users of the use of the cell phone. https://www.ncbi.nlm.nih.gov/pmc/articles/PMC5152665/

The precautionary principle was not observed in any way during the massive deployment of these wireless technologies.

However, when serious and possibly irreversible risks have been identified, uncertainty should not be used as a pretext to postpone measures to protect the environment and health.

We have reviewed the independent scientific literature and we refer, among other things, to Resolution 1815 of the Parliamentary Assembly of the Council of Europe. Our conclusions are in line with those of independent specialists, and that the precautionary principle does not currently apply and that the protection of the health of citizens, and of children in particular, is not guaranteed against overexposure to these electromagnetic radiation. RF / MO.

Standards intended to protect the population from exposure to RF / MO electromagnetic radiation only take into account tissue heating (thermal effect) during a limited duration exposure.

These standards do not take into account repeated and / or prolonged exposures, or the non-thermal biological effects that occur at values significantly lower than the currently authorized values. They were not designed to protect fetuses, children, adolescents, the elderly, etc.

For children, the risks may increase due to the cumulative effects of prolonged exposure. Your developing and immature brains, organs, and tissues may be more sensitive to exposure. And radiation penetrates proportionally more deeply into their organs than in adults since their dimensions are smaller.

The widespread deployment of wireless technologies has known health risks for several decades.

The absence of serious evidence, from independent scientific studies, that prove the safety in public health by radiation of frequency waves of cellular or mobile telephone technology and 5G technology.

On the other hand, there are several international associations that have sufficient evidence of what has caused physical and psychological injuries to people by radiation of frequency waves from cell phone or mobile technology and 5G.

Study that should be done in all cities by INDEPENDENT organisms and revised as it says here the radiation level to adapt it to the scientifically proven health impacts

High ambient radiofrequency

radiation in the city of Stockholm (Sweden)
2019 doi: 10.3892 / ol. 2018.9789

We measured radio frequency (RF) radiation in the central parts of Stockholm, Sweden, in March and April 2017. The same measurement path was used each time. We use EME Spy 200 for measurements as in our previous studies in Stockholm. Results were based on 11,482 entries, corresponding to more than 12 h of measurements. The total mean level was 5,494 μW / m2 (median 3,346; range 36.6–205,155). The main contributions were downlinks from LTE 800 (4G), GSM + UMTS 900 (3G), GSM 1800 (2G),

UMTS 2100 (3G) and LTE 2600 (4G). Regarding the different locations, the highest RF radiation was measured in the Hay Market with an average level of 10,728 µW / m2 (median 8,578; range 335-68,815). This is a plaza used for shopping, and both retailers and visitors can spend considerable time here. Furthermore, the Sergel Plaza had high radiation with an average of 7,768 µW / m2. All measurements exceeded the target level of 30–60 µW / m2 based on non-thermal effects (no heating), according to the BioInitiative Report. Based on short-term thermal effects, the International

Commission for Protection against Non-Ionizing Radiation established guideline 2 of 10 W / m2 (2,000,000–10,000,000 μW / m2) depending on the frequency in 1998, and has not changed it despite solid evidence of thermal biological effects at substantially lower exposure levels. These levels of ambient RF radiation are expected to increase with the introduction of 5G for wireless communication. (Note: BioIniciative in a later review further lowers the healthy level of radiation. Very little radiation is needed to have mobile coverage!)
https://www.ncbi.nlm.nih.gov/p

mc/articles/PMC6341832/

Mobile phone microwave emissions exceed safety limits

In his Scientific guide from early 2019, Prof. Om. P. Gandhi shows that mobile phones do not meet the specific absorption rate (SAR) safety limits in both Europe and the US. USA He recommends that regulators change current compliance testing methods. As consumers, we generally think that all the electronic products we use, including mobile phones, are safe to use. When it comes to mobile phones and other wireless technologies, one of the security tests a product needs to pass before it is released to the market is a Specific Absorption Rate (SAR) test. The results of this test reveal whether the product is above or below an established safety limit. Professor Gandhi reveals that current safety standards and the way these tests are performed do not provide true results for us consumers. And because of that, we cannot trust them. We will explain why.

What is SAR?

To make it as simple as
possible, the SAR is a value
set in W / kg that gives you
an idea of how much
radiation it absorbs while
making a phone call (with a
phone on your head),
downloading files, or
connecting to Wi-Fi .

What is wrong with current
SAR testing methods?

Unrealistic distance between
phone and body:

According to the professor, in
the last 5-10 years,
manufacturers began to
recommend that we hold a
phone between 5 and 25 mm
from the body. The same is

done with SAR tests.
But what if we do the same tests at a distance of 0 mm from the body, the way we usually use a phone?

The vast majority of people usually carry a phone in their pocket or body, or place it directly on their ear when they answer a call (i.e. unless they use a speakerphone or headphones). When we surf, we usually carry a phone in one hand.

It has already been shown that the closer the phone is to the body, the higher the SAR reading will be.

That is why Professor Gandhi believes that without

adding distance as part of the established test conditions, most wireless devices will not comply.

SAR measurements at different distances

To illustrate your point, take a look at the following SARs in W / kg measured for representative phones (out of the 450 tested). They were held against the flat phantom model of the body at distances suggested by the manufacturer (D) and at distances of 5 and 0 mm. (Table taken from reference 1):

The results clearly show that at a distance of 0mm, none of the tested phones exceeds the current safety limit of 2W / kg in Europe and 1.6 (W / kg) in the US. USA

Realistic head / body model:

Professor Gandhi confirms that the current test model is based on an oversized head army recruitment test model. Based on this, it is only clear that such a baseline is not adequate to reflect the variety of phone users. What about SAR in children with a much thinner skull and who develop the brain, or in women and men with smaller heads?

Recommendation: change current test conditions

Professor Gandhi strongly suggests that industry regulators establish compliance testing under realistic conditions. He recommends that:
Test at 0mm distance to reflect a realistic user experience
Include a variety of phantom models to include smaller headed boys, women, and men.

What do you get out of this?

Now that you have been educated on how things work behind the scenes of mobile phone security testing, we sincerely hope

that you use your critical
thinking and common sense
and remember that:
A lower SAR rating does not
necessarily make a phone
safer for everyday use.
Unless your head is the same
size as that of a 100g army
recruit, it will always
absorb a greater amount of
radiation.
Children absorb much more
radiation than adults.

We do not ask you to stop
using your phone and other
wireless devices suddenly.
But we invite you to take
good care of your body to
build resilience and limit
exposure whenever
possible.

References

https://ieeexplore.ieee.org/stamp/stamp.jsp?tp=&arnumber=8688629

https://ehtrust.org/new-study-cell-phones-exceed-safety-limits-when-phones-touch-the-body /

https://ieeeaccess.ieee.org/?http://ieeeaccess_ieee_org/

https://www.pewresearch.org/global/2019/02/05/smartphone-ownership-is- growing-rapidly-around-the-world-but-not-always-alike /

Why should you turn off the wifi at night?

How many of you are sleeping with the phone next to your head and the wifi constantly on?
Have you ever thought that turning off the wifi at night could be part of the solution and improve the health of your family?
Electromagnetic fields (EMF), also called radio frequency.

Since Wi-Fi is one of the main sources of EMF in your home, turning it off at night could be a simple step to help you sleep better and reduce your exposure by a third.

Let us explain why.

If you're new to the topic of radio frequencies, microwave radiation, and EMFs, start with our article titled "The Beginner's Guide to Electromagnetic Radiation."

Done?

Next, let's answer the main question and take a look at the Bioinitiative report on the effects of EMF on health. Compiled by 29 independent scientists and health experts from around the world, this report is just one of many reliable resources available online that show evidence of the effects and potential risks of wireless technologies and electromagnetic fields.

According to this report, the bioeffects (effects on human, animal or cellular biology) are clearly established and take place at very low levels of exposure to electromagnetic fields and radiofrequency radiation, either through the use of a mobile or wireless phone,

Mobile phone masts, WI-FI and "smart" wireless utility meters that produce full body exposure.

Studies cited in the report show that these exposures can not only cause DNA damage, but can also cause oxidative stress (think faster about aging and disease) and can be carcinogenic. Studies have also been conducted showing the impact on sperm function, the brain, and the nervous system, as well as behavior in offspring.

Therefore, the more we are exposed to these fields and wireless radiation, the more the body needs to keep up to date and control everything and combat this source of stress.

This is exactly the reason why turning off your wifi overnight is one of the simplest things to help combat the EMF problem. It is not the only solution, but reducing the exposure time by 7 or 8 hours a day, whenever possible, is definitely worth it.

Top 5 tips to help you sleep like a baby

Have you ever been around and around in your bed, unable to calm your mind until the wee hours of the morning? Have you ever stayed up late looking at a computer screen for hours only to find it difficult to fall asleep immediately afterward?

If you said yes to any of the above, read on. We've compiled 5 top tips to help you sleep better, get enough rest, and wake up more alert and ready for the day ahead.

Why is high-quality sleep one of the secrets to a healthier life?

Sleep is one of the vital components of life. During the ideal sleep of 7 to 9 hours (recommended for adults) your body rests and regenerates. Your organs, muscles, and cells recover and repair. Your brain can process and remove the accumulation of metabolic waste from the day and create new connections and memories.

Lack of sleep and poor sleep quality have been linked to mood and attention problems, irritability, anxiety, premature aging, and even Alzheimer's disease.

What impacts your dream?

Here is a list of the top eight
   factors that may be
   influencing your sleep.

Electromagnetic frequencies
   (EMF) of wireless devices
   and dirty electricity

Not sure what EMFs are?
   Learn about them in our
   article "The Beginner's
   Guide to Electromagnetic
   Radiation." (link to blog
   post)
If you do Knod, did you know
   that wireless radiation has
   been shown to harm sleep
   and affect the brain?
   According to the
   Environmental Health
   Trust, it could lead to an
   increased toxic load on the

body.

Wireless device EMFs have also been found to delay the so-called non-REM deep sleep stage and shorten the time spent there. Non-REM deep sleep is a state in which your body repairs itself, builds tissues, and strengthens the immune system, making it crucial for your body to receive it.

But that is not all. So-called "dirty electricity" or low-frequency electromagnetic fields emitted by electrical circuits and plugs could play a role in affecting your heart rate.

Because we at Qi-Technologies are experts in helping you solve problems related to the effects of electromagnetic radiation from wireless devices, we have gone further in explaining how wireless devices that emit electromagnetic radiation can affect your sleep (link to name and article here to come))

Light

Light affects your brain directly through special light-sensitive cells in our eyes, which decide whether it is day or night.

Too many hours in front of a screen can significantly influence your sleep cycle and have a greater impact on your sleep.

Shift work and travel

Light changes due to a change
   in work hours or when
   traveling through time
   zones strongly influence our
   internal clock and our
   ability to sleep at various
   times.

Stress, pain, anxiety, and
   other medical conditions.

If you are constantly under
   psychological, emotional, or
   physical stress, you may
   find it difficult to fall
   asleep. Pain can also cause
   light or interrupted sleep.

Medicines, coffee, alcohol and
   other substances.

Caffeine, alcohol, nicotine,
   antihistamines, as well as

certain prescription medications that include beta-blockers, alpha-blockers, and antidepressants, can affect sleep quality.

The foods you eat

The foods you eat (including drinks) will help healthy sleep on the contrary. Highly processed foods with high sugar / carbohydrate content will affect the way your body relaxes for sleep. The sugar in your system is able to get you out of a deep sleep, making you feel easily exhausted the next day.

Exercise

According to the US National Sleep Foundation. In the USA, less time sitting is associated with better sleep and health, and exercising at any time of the day appears to be good for sleeping.

The environment in which you sleep

The light, noise, temperature and quality of the mattress / bed mentioned above can affect the way you sleep. There is no prescribed sleeping temperature, but a little

The colder environment generally works better.

Extreme temperatures in sleeping environments tend to disrupt sleep.

What can you do to sleep better?

Here are 5 simple steps to help you recharge your sleep.
Limit EMF exposure when possible

If possible, turn off the fuse in your room to decrease low-frequency EMFs.
Turn off the wifi at night. Find out why you need to turn off your wifi at night (link to article)
Remove your phone and any wireless devices from your room and your children's room at night.

If you're concerned about your children's sleep habits, you might like our article titled How EMFs Affect Children's Health (link).

Create a good sleep routine

Your routine may include going to bed at the same time every night, waking up at the same time every morning.
Relax by doing something relaxing, like bathing, gentle yoga, stretching, or reading.
Pick up a book or e-reader similar to paper without a backlight.

Create a nutritious environment

Keep your room tidy and
  clutter-free. When our
  brain is surrounded by
  disorder, it can be more
  difficult to calm down.
Use dim lights before turning
  off at night.
Open the window and let the
  air circulate.
Sleep in a dark room and keep
  the light off while sleeping.
Avoid looking at screens at
  night.

Reduce stress and stay fit

Stress keeps your body in a
  fight or flight mode and
  doesn't allow it to fully
  reset.
Find strategies to help you be
  more resilient and deal with
  stress more effectively on

a daily basis. This could include exercise, yoga, tai chi, meditation, mindfulness, developing more self-awareness, or regular massages.

Avoid heavy meals and caffeine.

Eliminate caffeine after noon and opt for a light dinner, ideally three hours before bed.
Skip sugary foods late at night to allow the body to rest. Now all you have to do is sleep like a baby!

References

https://ehtrust.org/key-issues/the-environment-and-health/wirelessradiationelectromagnetic-fields-increases-toxic-body-load /

https://ehtrust.org/key-issues/cell-phoneswireless/screens-and-sleep/

https://ehtrust.org/science/research-on-wireless-health-effects/

https://science.sciencemag.org/content/342/6156/373

https://www.sleep.org/articles/how-sleep-adds-muscle/

https://www.healthline.com/health/sleep-deprivation/effects-on-body#1

http://healthysleep.med.harvard.edu/healthy/science/how/external-factors

https://www.sleepscore.com/eat-well-sleep-well-how-diet-affects-your-sleep/

https://www.sleep.org/articles/sugar-impacts-sleep/

https://www.sleepfoundation.org/articles/5-facts-about-sleep-and-exercise

https://www.sleep.org/articles/easy-ways-to-create-a-soothing-bedroom-environment /

https://www.ncbi.nlm.nih.gov/pubmed/9258703

How does blue light affect your sleep?

Have you ever found yourself looking at a computer screen for hours, working, studying, browsing or watching a movie? You would stay up late, only to find yourself completely open as soon as your head hits the pillow.

Although there are some key things that can affect the quality of your sleep (blog link), the amount of time you spend using your wireless devices is one of the main influences on how well you will sleep.

And it is mainly due to blue light.

What is blue light?

It is fair to say that sunlight
is the main natural source
of blue light, which helps us
stay awake and alert during
the day.
On the other hand,
fluorescent and LED
lighting, flat-screen TV
screens, smartphone
screens, tablets, computers
are artificial devices that
also emit blue light.
According to Dr. Heiting,
Doctor of Optometry
(D.O.), although the amount
of blue light emitted by
these devices is only a
fraction of that emitted by
the sun, it is the amount

of the time we spend using
them and how close we are

to the screens that can
have possible long-term
effects on our health.

The body's biological clock:
    the circadian rhythm
Imagine that your body has a
    biological clock running on a
    24-hour cycle. Called the
    circadian rhythm or
    circadian clock, this
    biological clock controls
    your sleep-wake cycle.
Your eyes help you recognize
    where you are currently in
    the sleep-wake cycle. They
    react to exposure to light,
    including blue light, through
    light-sensitive cells.
At night, the eyes tell the
    brain that it is time to
    sleep and regenerate.

Darkness also causes the body
to produce a hormone called
"melatonin". This hormone,
produced in the pineal gland
of our brain, signals the
body to prepare for sleep.
In addition to this,
melatonin has antioxidant
and anti-inflammatory
properties and contributes
to healthy function of the
body's immune and
neurological system.
How does blue light impact
your sleep?

The blue light keeps you more
alert and awake and tricks
the body into thinking it is
still daylight. The body
clock is now shifted and out
of sync, causing him trouble
falling asleep, not getting

deep enough sleep, and waking up tired.

As a result, the body produces little or no melatonin overnight.

A 2014 study by researchers at Harvard Medical School in Boston showed that reading a backlit device before bed worsens your sleep significantly more than reading a paper book in low light.
The study reported that people who used an iPad at night:

It produced 55% less melatonin;
It took them an extra 10 minutes to fall asleep
I had less REM (Rapid Eye

Movement) sleep at night, which is when we dream. Waking up the next day, iPad readers felt more sleepy and took longer to feel alert compared to book readers.

Interestingly, the following night, the circadian clocks of iPad readers were delayed more than 90 minutes and their bodies began to feel tired an hour and a half later than normal.

What happens when you don't sleep?

Not giving your body the vital rest it needs can cause all kinds of problems.

Lack of sleep prevents your brain from releasing toxins accumulated during waking hours.

A recent study led by researchers at the University of Washington School of Medicine in St. Louis, MO, suggests that adults who don't get enough sleep may be on their way to developing Alzheimer's disease.

Lack of sleep can cause memory problems, concentration problems, or mood swings. It can also weaken your immune system, increase inflammation and the risk of type 2 diabetes.

Improve your sleep hygiene for better health

It is now clear how important sleeping is and why you should reduce your exposure to blue light at night. Here are 5 tips to get there:

Use filters and blue light blockers on your devices. It will help you reduce exposure to artificial blue light during the day.

Stop any activity on your mobile devices and computers at least 2-3 hours before bed. Allow your body to begin preparing for sleep.

Dims the lights at night. Turn off the LED lights and choose a softer, orange and yellow light to reduce exposure to blue light.

How to read? Opt for a backlit paperless e-book or e-reader.

Turn off the wifi and remove your phone and any wireless devices from your room overnight. Wireless devices emit electromagnetic radiation that can also affect your sleep.

References

https://www.medicalnewstoday.com/articles/324161.php
https://www.healthline.com/health/sleep-deprivation/effects-on-body#1
https://www.allaboutvision.com/cvs/blue-light.htm
https://www.sleepfoundation.o

rg/articles/me brass-and-sleep
https://www.pnas.org/content/112/4/1232
https://www.researchgate.net/publication/272518070_Antioxidant_Properties_of_Melatonin_and_its_Potential_Action_in_Diseases
https://ehtrust.org/key-issues/cell-phoneswireless/screens-and-sleep/

The Beginner's Guide to Electromagnetic Radiation

What do a rainbow, a mobile phone and a CT scan of the head have in common?

One thing is for sure. They all emit EMFs (electromagnetic fields), or else they are called electromagnetic radiation (EM radiation).

We often talk about EM radiation in connection with mobile phones and cables. EM radiation includes much more than this.

We will explain some very basic concepts to help you understand where wireless technology fits:

What is EM radiation?

What is the EM spectrum?

What types of EM radiation
are there?
What is ionizing and non-
ionizing radiation?
What are the health effects
of EM radiation?

What is electromagnetic
radiation?

When you sit in a car to drive
to your favorite theater, it
takes you there because its
motor creates enough
energy to make it move.
When we speak of
movement, we speak of
"kinetic energy".
By nature, EM radiation is also
a form of energy. Let's
take a look at how
everything works.

While using your car to travel

where you want to be, EM radiation uses an "electrically charged particle" as a vehicle.
And depending on its qualities, this particle could travel through the air, through any matter, including the human body, the concrete walls or even the vacuum.
As the electrically charged particle travels, it disrupts the environment around it through "electromagnetic waves."

What is the electromagnetic spectrum?

Not all EM radiation is created equal. So what makes one type of EM radiation different from another?

They behave differently
depending on the quality of
the waves they create,
what we call "wavelength"
or "frequency".
To illustrate this, imagine two
ships traveling across the
ocean. The first pot is
three times bigger than the
other. Will the waves
created by both ships in
the surrounding waters be
exactly the same?
No, he will not. The size and
frequency of the waves will
depend on the size of the
boat and the speed (energy)
it is using to move forward.
The same applies to
wavelength and frequency.

Electromagnetic waves with
higher energy and
frequency are shorter,

while waves with lower
energy and frequencies are
longer.
On the basis of these
characteristics we can
organize them in the
electromagnetic spectrum
(EM).

Source:
https://marine.rutgers.edu
/cool/education/class/josh/
em_spec.html

What types of EM radiation
are there?

We can group certain
frequency ranges into
different types, from the
lowest wavelengths to the
highest and the amount of
energy they carry:

Source: https:
//www.mirion.com/learning-
center/radiation-safety-
basics/what-is- radiation

Power lines

Power lines have the lowest
wavelengths.

Radio waves

Radio waves are transmitted
by radio broadcasts,
television broadcasts,
radars, and even mobile
phones.

Some examples of radio
spectrum bands include
Extremely Low Frequency
(ELF), Ultra Low Frequency
(ULF), Low Frequency (LF),
Medium Frequency (MF),

Ultra High Frequency (UHF), and Extremely High Frequency (EHF).

Bluetooth, Wi-Fi, cordless phones, GPS, and 5G use the ultra-high frequency ranges. 5G will also use the extremely high frequency range.

Microwave

Microwaves can be used to transmit information through space, as well as to heat food. Some of the 5G frequencies will be in the microwave range.

Infrared radiation

Infrared radiation can be released as heat or thermal

energy. Infrared cameras, for example, would use this radiation to detect heat.

Visible light

Visible light is the only part of the electromagnetic spectrum that humans can see. Rainbow colors would fall in the visible spectrum of electromagnetic radiation, and each color would have its own wavelength.

Ultraviolet light

UV light is responsible for your tan or sunburn.

X-rays

Unlike light, X-rays have

higher energy and can pass through most objects, including the body. They are commonly used in medical X-rays, mammograms, CT scans, fluoroscopy, and in radiation therapy (cancer treatments).

Gamma rays

Gamma rays are generated by radioactive atoms and in nuclear explosions.

Ionizing versus non-ionizing radiation

ER radiation can also be divided into two groups depending on the severity of the radiation. Ionizing radiation contains a large amount of energy to remove electrons and cause atoms to decompose.

Higher frequency waves, such as X-rays and gamma rays, have ionizing radiation.

Low frequency waves, like radio waves, do not have ionizing radiation and are grouped together as non-ionizing.

What are the health effects of EM radiation?

The fact that radiation is not ionizing does not mean that it does not affect our biology.

EM radiation emitted by mobile phones, wifi routers,

and similar wireless devices has had biological effects on our cells, including increased inflammation and oxidative stress, fertility, or cognitive function.
You can read the following articles related to this topic (link to all articles):

"Are all EMFs harmful?"
How do EMFs affect children's health? 5G: Is your family's health at risk?
What is the Mobile Phone's Specific Absorption Rate (SAR) ?: Health and Safety Concerns Mobile phone emissions exceed safety limits

Resources:

https://www.medicalnewstoday.com/articles/219970.php
https://www.livescience.com/50326-what-is-ultraviolet-light.html
https://chem.libretexts.org
https://marine.rutgers.edu/cool/education/class/josh/em_spec.html
https://www.nibib.nih.gov/science-education/science-topics/x-rays
https://www.lifewire.com/5g-spectrum-frequencies-4579825
The World Health Organization (WHO), IARC classifies radio frequency electromagnetic fields as possibly carcinogenic to humans. Press release, May 31, 2011.

http://www.iarc.fr/en/medi
a-
centre/pr/2011/pdfs/pr20
8_E.pdf
https://www.who.int/peh-
emf/about/WhatisEMF/en/

Are all electromagnetic fields
(EMF) harmful?

Interested in keeping your
family healthy? If so,
chances are you have come
across the term "EMF"
(electromagnetic fields),
specifically in relation to
mobile phones, wifi routers,
laptops or smart meters.
Due to its unfavorable
impact on our well-being,
the reputation that EMFs
have earned is very
negative.

But are they all the same? Are they all harmful? The answer is no. They are not

Certain types of electromagnetic fields occur naturally and are an integral part of life on Earth as we know it. And the specific types of EMF can even be used therapeutically, for example, to speed up the healing of broken bones.

In the following lines we will explain:

What are electromagnetic fields?
How do they occur in nature?
What's the problem with man-made mobile phone EMFs?
How to protect your family

from harmful EMFs?

What are electromagnetic fields?

Essentially, we are all born in the sea from electromagnetic fields. Like the gravitational forces that keep our feet on the ground, electromagnetic fields are one of the fundamental forces in nature.

They are basically a combination of electric and magnetic fields and come in different "shapes and sizes".

In the image below, you can see that they differ in their wavelength (how far between each wave) and frequency (how fast the wave changes). On the basis of these characteristics we can organize them into a so-called electromagnetic spectrum (EM).

Ionizing versus non-ionizing radiation

The EM spectrum includes both ionizing and non-ionizing radiation ranges. Ionizing radiation is a type of electromagnetic field that carries enough energy to break down molecules (ionization atoms) and can be deadly. Examples include X-rays, gamma rays, and various types of radioactive materials.

On the other hand, non-ionizing radiation does not carry enough energy to break molecular bonds. Power lines, microwaves, radio waves, infrared radiation, visible light, and lasers are examples of this type of EMF.

Source: https://ehtrust.org/wp-content/uploads/2015/12/Dr-Devra-Davis-Melb-Uni-Lecture.pdf

EMF: a brief explanation for the most technical

Electromagnetic fields are basically physical fields produced by electrically charged objects. They are able to influence the behavior of other charged objects in their vicinity and can be seen as the combination of an electric and magnetic field. The

electric field is produced
by stationary charges
(without flux) and the
magnetic field by mobile
charges (currents).
An electromagnetic field is
defined by its frequency
and wavelength. The
frequency and wavelength
of the field are directly
related to each other: the
higher the frequency, the
shorter the wavelength.

How do EMFs occur in nature?

Credits: Peter Reid
    (peter.reid@ed.ac.uk), 2009
Source:
    https://www.nasa.gov/topic
    s/earth/features/2012-
    poleReversal.html

In addition to some of the examples mentioned , there are more sources of electric, magnetic and electromagnetic fields as we find them in nature. Many of them are not harmful to life:

We see electrical fields produced by the local accumulation of electrical charges, such as s in the atmosphere associated with electrical storms.

Animals, like birds or fish, use Earth's magnetic field for navigation. A compass needle does the same thing when moving in a north-south direction.

Your body creates its own electromagnetic field (we are all made of atoms!). It is the only way it can exist

as a single entity.
Light and colors are part of
    the natural electromagnetic
    spectrum.
Ultraviolet light from the sun.

EMF sources made by man

The ability to listen to your
    favorite radio station, use a
    mobile phone, watch TV,
    connect to Wi-Fi, or use an
    x-ray to diagnose a broken
    bone - these are all
    examples of artificial EMF
    in action.

Even the electricity that
    powers our house, for
    example, is associated with
    EMF at a very low
    frequency.

Source:
https://ehtrust.org/wp-content/uploads/2015/12/Dr-Devra-Davis-Melb-Uni-Lecture.pdf

What is the problem with human created EMFs from cell phones, towers or wifi routers?

Dr. Devra Davis, president of the Environmental Health Trust, explains that the impact of any form of EMF depends on the nature of the waves they emit. The nature of microwaves that telephones, telephone masts, wifi, and similar technologies is pulsed, erratic, and highly irregular.

Imagine your cells "listening"
and responding to this pulse
for thousands of minutes
per month, for many hours
a week, throughout life.
How does your body feel?

The truth is that our body
does not have the
mechanisms to adapt to
such explosions of an
irregular signal. And it's
also difficult to know what
dose of this pulsed signal
your body is receiving at
any time, depending on
where you are.

According to Dr. Beverly
Rubik, a biophysicist and
researcher, experiencing
this over and over again can
have a cumulative effect,
which in some cases leads

to electrosensitivity.

And research already suggests
some disturbing effects on
this type of EMF, including
an increased risk of
infertility, neurological
problems, increased
inflammation, or cancer.

How to protect your family
from harmful EMFs?

Doctors, surgeons and
biomedical scientists from
the Global Campaign for
Safer Cell Phones
recommend:
Do not hold the phone directly
against your head or body -
use a speaker or other
hands-free device.
Use landline phone: wired
landlines are safer.

Cordless phones emit
microwave radiation.

Watch out for a weak signal:
    Your phone has to work
    harder and emit more
    radiation when the signal is
    weak or blocked.
Protect children and the
    pregnant abdomen: Children
    absorb twice as much
    radiation as adults.
Men who want to become
    fathers: beware: sperm are
    especially vulnerable to
    radiation.
Do not send text messages
    while on the move: p.
    driving, cycling, skating,
    walking, skiing. Milliseconds
    can make the difference
    between life or death.
You can also choose to use
    protective materials in your

home, such as protective curtains or wall paints, or use a Qi-Home cell (link to store) to protect your home from EMFs.

Resources:

Rubik B. (2014). Does short-term exposure to cell phone radiation affect blood? The Wise Traditions in Food, Agriculture and the Healing Arts, Vol. 15 (4), pp 19-28.
http://www.westonaprice.org/modern-diseases/does-short-term-exposure-to-cell-phone-radiation-affected-the-blood /
https://www.iarc.fr/wp-content/uploads/2018/07/pr208_E.pdf
The World Health Organization (WHO), IARC

classifies radio frequency electromagnetic fields as possibly carcinogenic to humans. Press release, May 31, 2011.
http://www.iarc.fr/en/media-centre/pr/2011/pdfs/pr208_E.pdf
https://www.who.int/peh-emf/about/WhatisEMF/en/
Non-thermal biological effects of
Microwave https://pdfs.semanticscholar.org/d87e/c3986fc706ef05926a609b3bf709872dd15e.pdf
Wireless World of Communications and Our Health - Beverly Rubik, PhD (2015) https://www.youtube.com/watch?v=K_RwRpfimfk (watch

about 7 minutes -
electromagnetic spectrum)
https://www.ntia.doc.gov/files
/ntia/publications/2003-
allochrt.pdf
https://www.iarc.fr/wp-
content/uploads/2018/07/p
r208_E.pdf
https://ehtrust.org/resources
-to-share/printable-
resources /? mgi_195 =
6570 / doctors-advice-on-
cell-phones-brochure

https://www.forbes.com/sites
/quora/2017/11/03/how-
the-human-body-creates-
electromagnetic-fields / #
6b1feff756ea
https://ehtrust.org/wp-
content/uploads/2015/12/D
r-Devra-Da vis-Melb-Uni-
Lecture.pdf

5G: Is your family's health at risk?

In this article we want to help you clearly understand:

What is 5G and why do we have to talk about it?
Are there any health risks that we should be aware of?
What can you do with 5G?

What is 5G?

5G is the fifth generation wireless network. From upgrade from 1st (1G) to 3rd and 4th generation (4G), you can enjoy the mobile phone experience of calling, texting, sending images, downloading data and surfing the Internet faster than ever. 5G goes beyond that.

The telecommunications industry convinces us that this "5G" will bring us closer together, offering complete interconnectivity, the future with autonomous cars and smart appliances. Our children's education face will be transformed with data speeds and responsiveness nearly 1,000% faster than 4G.

Germany aims for full 5G connectivity by 2025 with Deutsche Telekom having started the first launch of the 5G network in March 2019.

There are currently 215,619 cell towers in Germany (according to Cellmapper, cell towers and coverage mapping service) excluding 5G. This will increase by 300 5G towers during 2019 alone.

In April 2019, Swisscom began operating with the first operational 5G network in Switzerland with estimated completion and full coverage before the end of 2019.

The United States is following the "5G FAST Plan" to make the United States the leader in 5G technology. Eight mobile network operators, including g Verizon, T-Mobile and

AT&T already offer 5G
mobile services in select
cities across the country.

Exciting, isn't it?
So it was during the 19040s
    and 50s when the tobacco
    industry did a great job of
    marketing cigarettes as
    perfect for perfect health.
    However, many lives lost
    afterward, lung cancer
    rates proved that we were
    all wrong.

What if history repeats
    itself?

The international appeal of
    EMF scientists

As of June 15, 2019, 248 EMF
    (electromagnetic field)
    scientists from 42 nations

have signed the ``
International EMF
Scientists Appeal '',
urgently calling on the
United Nations and its sub-
organizations, WHO and
UNEP, and all UN Member
States, Greater protection
of health from exposure to
EMF.

They unanimously share their
concern about the global
public health crisis thanks
to increasing levels of
environmental pollution
from infrastructure and
electrical and wireless
devices.

The late Dr. Martin Blank
(1933-2018), an EMF
expert who originally
announced the Appleal in
2015, shares a compelling
message on behalf of the

signatories:
Download the transcript of your message.

Other organizations, such as the Environmental Health Trust and the Physician's Health Initiative for Radiation Protection (PHIRE) do the same, warning us about the effects and risks of EMF, including 5G.

4G vs 5G

The 5G network will use everything 4G does. But there is more:
It will work in additional frequency ranges, including very high frequency millimeter waves (20-300 GHz), different modulation,

higher amplitude, and fast bursts of data.
You will need smaller, denser antennas (cell towers between 100m to several kilometers) to create better connectivity.
A 4G cell tower currently supports around 2,000 devices with some traffic delays. A 5G tower will support more than a million connected devices per square kilometer with negligible delays.

With these added "extras" we can be sure of one thing. More radiation for all living things.

5G: 10 risks you should know

If you are concerned about

your health and the health
of your loved ones, please
note that even 5G comes
with luggage:
Radio frequencies (RF or EMF)
can cause serious biological
effects, such as cancer,
alteration of the nervous
system or reproductive
deterioration. RF was
classified as a possible
Group 2B human carcinogen
by the World Health
Organization in 2011.

Children, pregnant women and
the elderly are more
vulnerable. (Read our blog
"The Effects of EMFs on
Children").

Your pets and wild animals can
be affected in the same
way as humans.

Solid research on higher
frequency millimeter waves
used by 5G is lacking.
PHIRE states that there is
evidence of biological
damage to humans, animals,
including insects and plants.

Greater numbers of cell
towers and transmitters
near living areas means
higher exposure rates.

If your child is bombarded by
a frequency "soup" now, the
long-term effects could
show up 20-30 years later,
when it is too late.

Higher frequency millimeter
waves are absorbed more
superficially. This raises a
matter of harmful effects

on human skin, eyes and testicles.

No one has given you, the public, an option to choose not to participate or sign an informed consent to be irradiated with radio frequencies (see www.5Gappeal.eu).

No safety limits are set to protect you against the non-thermal effects of EMFs.

The current EMF absorption rate safety limits do not reflect the way we use our phones (read our article "What is SAR?" And "Safety limits ...")

What can you do with 5G?

If you're concerned about
   EMFs and 5G, you have
   three options:

Raise awareness in your local
   community and share this
   article everywhere.
Join the 5G debate and
   educate yourself more with
   independent resources:
   Appel-de-paris.com
5Gappeal.eu Bioinitiative.org

Ehtrust.org Emfcall.org
   Emfscientist.org
   Mdsafetech.org Orsaa.org
   Phiremedical.org
   Radiationresearch.org
   Saferemr.com
Wirelessriskassessment.org

Resources:
http://www.bfs.de/EN/topics/

emf/mobile-
communication/basics/5g/5
g.html
https://www.electricsense.co
m/is-5g-dangerous/
https://tobaccocontrol.bmj.co
m/content/21/2/87
https://www.gettingsmart.com
/2019/04/5-ways-5g-will-
make-classrooms-smarter/
https://www.who.int/peh-
emf/meetings/archive/en/p
roceedings_eng.pdf
https://www.swisscom.ch/en/a
bout/company/portrait/net
work/5g.html
https://ehtrust.org/key-
issues/cell-
phoneswireless/5g-
internet-everything/20-
quick-facts-what-you-need-
to-know-about-5g-wireless-
and-small-cells /
https://www.telekom.com/en/

media/media-information/archive/deutsche-telekom- is-ready-to-launch-5g-in-germany-575974

https://www.cellmapper.net/networks?country=262&net=ALL

https://www.rcrwireless.com/20190708/5g/opensignal-us-has-the-fastest-5g-peak-speed

https://www.lifewire.com/5g-availability-us-4155914

https://www.fcc.gov/5G

https://www.lifewire.com/5g-news-4428066

https://www.dw.com/en/5g-auction-in-germany-raises-65-billion-from-four-telcoms / a-49168657

How EMFs Affect Children's Health

As parents, grandparents, aunts, uncles, friends, and guardians, we are responsible for ensuring that our children are healthy and thrive. With wireless technologies and devices all around us, we need to be well informed about safety and potential risks to protect the most vulnerable: our children.

In this article we will help you understand:

how microwave radiation, also called electromagnetic fields (EMF), emitted by wireless devices and mobile phones can be harmful to children's health

why children are more at risk

than adults
what evidence do we have to
   support this
How we can protect children
   from EMF at home

A baby and an iphone

Imagine this. A beautiful baby.
   It should be only a few
   weeks old. So fragile, with
   his cute little nose, soft
   cheeks and the smallest
   fingers. And an iPhone that
   plays relaxing music. Placed
   just a few inches from his
   small head.
How could this originally well-
   intentioned act of parental
   love, which I have
   witnessed, affect the
   baby's health?
If you want to know, keep
   reading.

Microwave radiation (EMF):
possible class 2B carcinogen
The World Health
Organization (WHO)
International Agency for
Research on Cancer (IARC)
has declared well-known
compounds such as
chloroform, DDT, lead,
nickel, gasoline and diesel
fuel as possible Class 2B
carcinogens.

We wouldn't dare think about
exposing a child to these
chemicals and we really
need to think the same way
about microwave radiation.
Since 2011, microwave
radiation is now also on the
list of possible Class B
carcinogens.
In 2014, researchers from the
Environmental Health Trust

and the University of California conducted a comprehensive review of peer-reviewed mobile phone exposure studies between 2009 and 2014. This review noted some troubling effects of microvawe radiation, including an increased risk of oxidation stress, brain cancer, and parotid gland tumors.

Do children absorb more microwave radiation than adults?
Multiple studies show that children absorb more radiation than adults for the following reasons:
his brain is more absorbing
their skulls are thinner
the size of her head is smaller.

Practically speaking, if my 4-year-old niece and I, a 36-year-old woman, talk to each other on the phone at the same time, she, a girl, will absorb at least two or three times. times more radiation than me, an adult.

Joe Wiart, principal investigator for French Telecom and Orange, confirmed this in a study published in 2008.

In 2010, another study by a research team at the Institute of Physics and Engineering in Medicine showed that children's bone marrow specifically absorbs 10 times more radiation than adults.

Other significant effects of EMFs on the children's brains:
Learning and memory deficiencies
Symptoms related to attention deficit hyperactivity disorder
Increased neural cell death.
Neural abnormalities and degeneration.

We discuss the effects of EMFs on brain function in more detail in our article titled "The Effects of EMFs on Brain Function" (link when ready).

Keeping Your Kids Safe From EMFs At Home: Top 10 Tips
It is almost impossible to completely avoid exposure to microwave radiation,

especially outside the home. With that said, there are still some beneficial things we can do to protect our children at home. Here are 10 helpful tips:

Keep overall exposure to mobile phones, WLAN routers, and baby monitors to a minimum.

Use phones and wireless devices with lower radiation / SAR values.

If you are using a baby monitor, place it as far away from the crib as possible. The Federal Office of Radiation Protection reports that baby monitors with rechargeable batteries emit less radiation than those with a power source.

Ban mobile phones in

children's rooms.
Use a corded landline phone
and avoid using cordless
phones.
If you use a cordless phone,
be sure to place it in the
hallway. Avoid such phones
in rooms at all costs.
Turn off your wifi and mobile
devices completely at night.
Have your children make calls
only when absolutely
necessary.
Use parental controls and
available apps, such as
FamilyTime, to limit the
time you spend on mobile
devices.
Educate your children about
EMFs. Have a conversation.
It is worth starting early.

References

https://www.youtube.com/watch?v=BwyDCHf5iCY

http://www.bfs.de/SharedDocs/Kurzmeldungen/BfS/EN/2013/09-11-childrens-health.html

http://www.bfs.de/EN/topics/emf/hff/effect/hff-established/hff-established.html

https://www.sciencedirect.com/science/article/pii/S2213879X14000583

https://www.ncbi.nlm.nih.gov/pubmed/16510956

https://www.sciencedirect.com/science/article/pii/S2213879X14000583

https://www.ncbi.nlm.nih.gov/pmc/articles/PMC5504984/

Both you and I are just two of the five billion mobile phone users out there. Our phones have become a daily necessity for us. Have you ever wondered how much radiation you absorb when you make a phone call, download a file, or just when you have a phone in your pocket? How safe is it? And how did SAR arise?

What is the specific absorption rate of the mobile phone, SAR?

SAR stands for Specific Absorption Rate and is defined as the power absorbed by tissue mass and has units of watts per kilogram (W / kg). What does it really mean?

Electromagnetic universe

Because we live in an electromagnetic (EM) universe (think light, color, infrared, all of which are part of the electromagnetic spectrum) we interact with a variety of EM sources every day.
Some of them are natural to the body and can be

beneficial to us. Others, although they occur naturally, can have harmful effects (think of sunburn). In addition to natural sources of EM waves, humanity was smart enough to create our own EM sources, to initially win our wars and finally take the human race to the next level of our evolution (think of mobile phones, Wifi, microwave).

What happens when you make a call?

When you make a call to your loved one, your phone (through its sophisticated antenna) intelligently sends your request (the information in the form of a signal) to a much stronger nearby tower. This tower then transmits this information, through the huge network of mobile masts, to the loved one of your choice.

Your body is a sponge

This invisible transmission signal is made of a type of energy, which we call radio frequency energy. It is measured in milliwatts (mW).

His body, on the other hand, is made up of biological tissues, the mass of which we measure in kilograms (kg).

In the process of connecting

and transmitting your call, the phone signal spreads in many directions. Most of this signal continues to the mobile tower, but some of it is absorbed by whatever is nearby. You, holding your phone by your head, become the "sponge" or "absorption pad" (in kg) of this energy.

How is SAR calculated?

When we measure SAR, the specific absorption rate, in fact, we calculate how much a part of this energy (in watts per kilogram) absorbs your body (biological tissues).
In more technical terms, it is the measurement of absorbed radio frequency (RF) energy in grams of

biological tissues when exposed to a radio frequency electromagnetic field.

Going back to the beginning, it could now be a little clearer what it means when we say that the SAR value is the power absorbed per tissue mass and has units of watts per kilogram (W / kg).

It is usually averaged over the entire body or over a volume of sample (usually 1 g or 10 g of tissue). The published SAR value is the maximum level measured in the body part (eg head) studied over the indicated volume or mass.

What is the SAR value in an adult?

The current SAR value, which is the maximum allowable exposure value, is 2W / kg in Europe and 1.6W / kg in the US. USA This applies to phone manufacturers by different regulatory bodies in Europe and the USA. USA Measurement is generally performed with a phantom head and body at a small distance (about 5mm).

Where do the current SAR standards come from?

The first security standards were established more than 20 years ago around 1997, when a typical mobile phone user was military, medical, or business. At the time it was believed that the only

thing to avoid was the warming effect.
In one of the original tests in 1989, the military used the head of a 220-lb (about 100-kg) man on 98% of his recruits. The standards they set were to avoid heating the subject's brain after a 6-minute phone call.

Are the current SAR standards sufficient?

Definitely not. Current standards can be a tool for judging whether the phone is "safe" under regulatory standards, but they do not accurately assess the full extent of how our health is affected.
Recently, Professor Gandhi from the University of

Utah reported [link to our blog post] that SARs in W / kg that when kept at zero body distance, the absorption rate was up to three times higher than the European limits approved and more up to 11 times above the US limit. USA

Here are more reasons why current standards are not enough:

SAR actually refers to thermal effects, but the vast majority of recorded biological effects of chronic lifetime exposure are not thermal.
A series of reported effects at SAR levels much lower than the current safety standard at over.

Not enough information was
   provided on the amount of
   RF exposure under real-life
   and real-use conditions.
   Laboratory-tested
   exposures are only short-
   term, generally a few
   minutes long.
It does not reflect the variety
   of head and body sizes.
   Most of the population has
   much smaller heads and
   bodies than the 100-kg
   male military recruit.

Radiation based on current use
   is much higher today than in
   the past.
Current laboratory tests do
   not include variations for
   critical energy absorption
   points.
Different laboratories can
   perform measurements at

different distances from
the body.

The nature of the mobile
phone signal is not taken
into account. Because it is
pulsed in nature, the
average power may remain
low, but individual signal
bursts can be very high.

A child's developing brain
absorbs much more than an
adult's brain. SAR value in
children vs adults.

How to reduce the SAR of
your phone?

Research shows that radio
effects or radio
frequencies have been
reported in SAR as low as
0.2W / kg after a two-hour
exposure. This means that
you will not be fully

protected from the effects of radio frequencies, even if your SAR phone claims to be well below the approved limit.

With that said, there are some helpful tips we can share with you for added security:

Reduce the amount of time you spend carrying your phone in your pockets or holding it in your hands.

Stop holding your phone by your ear when you call.

Opt for a hands-free option or wear headphones when making a call.

Choose a mobile phone with a lower SAR rating. This will not necessarily be the key to security, but it will still be useful.

Keep your phone away from your body when you are on wifi, access points or downloading data. During those times the SAR levels increase significantly.

Ask yourself: Do I really need to spend four hours (on average) a day on my phone? It's really necessary? Otherwise, just put your phone aside instead of constantly checking it.

Turn off your phone or use airplane mode when possible. Not only will it make you safer, I bet you will also become less distracting, more productive, and more focused on the task at hand.

References

Mobile phone users Statistics
https://www.statista.com/stat
  istics/330695/number-of-
  smartphone-users-
  worldwide /
Wikipedia: Specific absorption
  rate
  https://en.wikipedia.org/wi
  ki/Specific_absorption_rat
  e
https://www.fcc.gov/consumer
  s/guides/specific-
  absorption-rate-sar-cell-
  phones-what-it-means-you
http://www.bfs.de/EN/topics/
  emf/mobile-
  communication/mobile-
  communication_node.html
https://fcc.report/FCC-
  ID/BCG-E3175A/3547302
https://fcc.report/FCC-

ID/A3LSMG950F
https://ehtrust.org/wp-
content/uploads/2015/12/D
r-Devra-Davis-Melb-Uni-
Lecture.pdf
Dr. Devra Davis Melbern
University
Conference
https://www.youtube.com/w
atch?v=BwyDCHf5iCY
Davis, Devra. Disconnect: The
truth about cell phone
radiation, what the industry
is doing to hide it, and how.
West 26th Street Press.
Kindle version.

http://www.emfwise.com/SAR.
php
https://www.ncbi.nlm.nih.gov/p
mc/articles/PMC3672148/
https://ieeexplore.ieee.org/st
amp/stamp.jsp?tp=&arnumb
er=8688629

SCIENTIFIC DATA:

Sci Rep. 2015 December 9; 5: 18030. doi: 10.1038 / srep18030.

Efficient microwave structure resonance energy transfer to virus-confined acoustic vibrations.

The virus is known to resonate in microwave confined acoustic dipole mode of the same frequency. However, this effect was not considered in previous studies of virus-microwave interaction and prevention of microwave-based virus epidemics. Here we show that this resonant energy transfer effect from the microwave structure to the virus can be efficient enough that the virus in the air is inactivated at a reasonable microwave power density safe for the open public. We demonstrate this effect by measuring the residual viral infectivity of influenza A virus after illuminating microwaves with different frequencies and powers. We also established a theoretical model to estimate the microwave power threshold for virus inactivation and good agreement was obtained with the experiments. Such inactivation induced by the transfer of resonant energy to the structure is mainly through the physical fracture of the virus structure, which was confirmed by real-time reverse transcription

polymerase chain reaction. These results provide a pathway to establishing a new open public epidemic prevention strategy for airborne viruses.
https://www.ncbi.nlm.nih.gov/pubmed/?term=Efficient+Structure+Resonance+Energy+Transfer+from+Microwaves+to+Confined+Acoustic+Vibrations+in+Viruses

PATENT:
https://patents.google.com/patent/CN1315847A/en

Format: Summary

Occup Environ Med. July 2014; 71 (7): 514-22. doi: 10.1136 / oemed-2013-101754. Epub 2014 May 9.

Use of mobile phones and brain tumors in the CERENAT case-control study.

Coureau G1, Bouvier G2, Lebailly P3, Fabbro-Peray P4, Gruber A5, Leffondre K6, Guillamo JS7, Loiseau H8, Mathoulin-Pélissier S6, Salamon R9, Baldi I10.

Author information

Summary

The carcinogenic effect of radio frequency electromagnetic fields in humans remains controversial. However, it has been suggested that they may be involved in the etiology of some types of brain tumors.

OBJECTIVES

The objective was to analyze the association between exposure to mobile phones and primary tumors of the central nervous system (gliomas and meningiomas) in adults.

METHODS:

CERENAT is a multicentre case-control study carried out in four areas in France in 2004-2006. Data on the use of mobile phones was collected through a detailed questionnaire delivered in person. Conditional logistic regression for matching sets was used to estimate the adjusted ORs and 95% CIs.

RESULTS

A total of 253 gliomas, 194 meningiomas, and 892 paired controls selected from local electoral lists were analyzed. No association with brain tumors was observed when comparing regular mobile phone users with non-users (OR = 1.24, 95% CI 0.86 to 1.77 for gliomas, OR = 0.90, 95% CI 0.61 to 1.34 for meningiomas). However, the positive association was statistically significant in the heaviest users when considering the cumulative lifetime duration ($\geq$896 h, OR = 2.89; 95% CI 1.41 to 5.93 for gliomas; OR = 2.57; 95% CI : 1.02 to 6.44 for meningiomas) and number of calls for gliomas ($\geq$18,360 calls, OR = 2.10, 95% CI 1.03 to 4.31). The risks were greater for gliomas, temporary tumors, use of urban and occupational mobile phones.

CONCLUSIONS

These additional data support previous findings about a

possible association
between heavy cell phone
use and brain tumors.

Published by the BMJ
Publishing Group Limited.
For permission to use
(where not licensed under
license), visit
http://group.bmj.com/grou
p/rights-licensing/pe
rmissions.

KEYWORDS
Case-control studies;
Electromagnetic fields;
Glioma; Meningioma; Mobile
phone; Radio frequency
electromagnetic fields
REFERENCE:
https://www.ncbi.nlm.nih.go
v/pubmed/24816517
Taken together, our results
suggest that regular use of

a mobile phone is associated
with the location of the
glioma in the sense that
more gliomas occurred
closer to the ear on the
side of the head where the
mobile phone was reported
to have used more.
However, this trend was
unrelated to the amount of
mobile phone use, making
the observed association
less likely to be caused by a
relationship between mobile
phone use and cancer risk.
We cannot draw firm
conclusions about cause and
effect, but our approach
has several strengths
compared to traditional
epidemiological approaches.
Our results may have been
affected by recall bias on
the reported side of phone

use. However, it offers an alternative for future research related to the use of mobile phones.

REFERENCE:

https://www.ncbi.nlm.nih.gov/pmc/articles/PMC5152665/

https://www.ncbi.nlm.nih.gov/pmc/articles/PMC6254861/

https://www.researchgate.net/publication/298533689_International_Appeal_Scientists_call_for_protection_from_non-ionizing_electromagnetic_field_exposure

https://www.researchgate.net/publication/331661949_Comparing_DNA_Damage_Induced_by_Mobile_Telephony_and_Other_Types_of_Man-Made_Electromagnetic_Fields

https://www.saferemr.com/20
16/05/national-toxicology-
progam-finds-cell.html
http://peaceinspace.blogs.com
/files/5g-emf-hazards-dr-
martin-l.-pall-eu-emf2018-
6-11us3.pdf
https://www.researchgate.net
/publication/273150433_M
obile_phone_radiation_caus
es_brain_tumors_and_shou
ld_be_classified_as_a_pro
bable_human_carcinogen_2
A_Review
https://bittube.video/videos/
watch/90d29122-7813-
47f5-adba-
f13253c05cfb?fbclid=IwAR
2ce8hsJgzMsn87ZOZ73e9
U8JDz9rhAx4cmcJFOhFX
8RAIzkyIBqoZSfxs
https://magdahavas.com/
https://www.dsalud.com/repor
taje/los-danos-para-la-

salud-de-la-tecnologia-5g-
y-su-relacion-con-la-
pandemia/
https://www.jrseco.com/can-
cell-phone-radiation-cause-
cancer-yes-says-ntp-rat-
study/
https://www.ecoportal.net/pai
ses/efectos-salud-redes-
5g/
https://bioinitiative.org/resea
rch-summaries/

DOCUMENT WITH MORE
THAN 1500 PAGES ON
THE EFFECTS OF
RADIATION
https://bioinitiative.org/table
-of-contents/
https://www.dsalud.com/repor
taje/nuevas-pruebas-de-
que-las-antenas-de-
telefonia-son-peligrosas/
https://www.gigahertz.es/blog

/index.php?434-medicos-belgas-contra-el-5g-&fbclid=IwAR3YgBZc3SCpktc9kX9ixDVManSnO1CBQsCr3S5-vPRoWkfnuWFTqm9f0nw
https://www.cienciasinmiedo.es/b415/

(# 415). RADIATION ISSUED BY MOBILE EXCEEDS THE LEGAL LIMITS

[ARTICLE REVIEW] In this article published in IEEE Access, the author comments on some of the results of the Phonegate case, that is, the discovery that the radiation emitted by a large number of mobile phones exceeds the levels recommended by the laws of various countries. .

As we have commented on other occasions in this blog, the safety guidelines on microwave exposure are governed mainly by the proposals of two committees: In the United States by the IEEE (Institute of Electrical and Electronics Engineers), and in other countries (among they Spain), by the ICNIRP (International Committee for nonionizing radiation protection).

Both standards are not homogeneous. In fact, the IEEE proposes a maximum specific absorption rate (SAR) of 1.6 W / kg per 1g of tissue, while ICNIRP prescribes a maximum of 2.0 W / kg for every 10g of tissue. As the author indicates, this methodological difference of considering 1 g versus 10 g of tissue means that ICNIRP standards allow approximately radiation with an intensity between 2.5 and 3 times.

Those recommendations are for all parts of the body except for the extremities, where a maximum of 4 W / kg is allowed. However, what the industry is doing is recommending that the mobile be used between 5 and 25 mm away from the body to meet the standards.

This leads to two important questions: (1) which mobile phone user reads or heeds these recommendations; (2) how realistic is that safety distance in relation to the common use of the device. The author reproduces some of the results of the study carried out by the French National Agency (ANFR) in 2017, on the SAR of 450 mobile devices. Apart from verifying that the manufacturers specifications are met (the SAR at the recommended distance), the ANFR also measured at distances of 5 mm and 0 mm from the body, much more consistent with the common use of mobiles. The French Agency used the same methodology as ICNIRP, that is, measuring SAR in 10 g of tissue.

The first table shows the SAR values of the manufacturer

compared to those of the evaluation at 5 mm, and the percentage of absorption that is above (or below) the legal limits for body and extremities.

The second table shows the manufacturer's SAR values compared to the evaluation at 0 mm, and also the percentage of absorption that is above (or below) the legal limits for body and limbs.

Comments.

The results are quite clear; several of the analyzed devices exceed the legal limits for the exposure of the body to 5 mm, and all do it (some of them in more than 200%) when the mobile is at 0 mm. It is not only necessary to consider these facts to make the pertinent legislative decisions, but also to assess to what extent future judicial disputes of patients who sue these companies may be conditioned.

It is true that the SAR for the extremities does not exceed 5 mm, but it does exceed 0 mm, which is precisely what happens when we have the mobile in hand. Furthermore, as the author indicates, when transferring these results to the 1 g tissue method used by the IEEE, a multiplying factor of 2.5 to 3 would have to be used, which would make them not comply at all with the limits proposed in countries such as, for example, example,

United States.

Therefore, not only do you have to worry about the possible consequences of prolonged exposure to microwaves (non-thermal effects), but also because, in many cases, the devices do not even meet the recommended levels to avoid thermal effects.

(# 256). MOBILE AND WI-FI INCREASE ANTIBIOTIC RESISTANCE

The E coli bacteria showed greater antimicrobial resistance to exposure to non-ionizing electromagnetic radiation and below legal limits during different time periods.

[ARTICLE REVIEW] There is research showing that electromagnetic fields can

affect cell growth and
antimicrobial susceptibility.
This last fact reflects, for
example, the resistance
capacity of bacteria against
antibiotics.

The authors focus this study
on the analysis of two
bacteria, Listeria
mocnocytogenes and
Echechichia coli, better
known as E coli. The first is
related to infections in
neonates or meningitis. The
second with infections in
the blood, urinary tract,
otitis and others.

The objective of this research
is to evaluate the
resistance to antibiotics of
these two bacteria in the
face of exposure to
radiofrequency
electromagnetic fields,

from two sources of different frequencies, 900 MHz and 2.4 GHz, corresponding to the signal of a GSM mobile phone and a Wi-Fi router, respectively.

Methodology

The bacteria were isolated after being collected from patients in an Iran hospital. A Mueller-Hinton agar compound containing 1.5 x 10 ^ 8 CFU / ml was created as a colony forming unit. That compound was dispersed in a container and treated with different antibiotics. For E coli imipenem (10 micrograms), levofloxacin (5 micrograms), aztreonam (30 micrograms), ciprofloxacin (5 micrograms), cefotaxime

(30 micrograms) and piperazillin (100 micrograms) were used. For listeria, doxycycline (30 micrograms), trimethoprim-sulfamethoxazole (25 micrograms), levofloxacin (5 micrograms), cefotaxime (30 micrograms), ciprofloxacin (5 micrograms) and cefriazone (30 micrograms) were used. The results of the bacteria's susceptibility to these antibiotics were measured before and after exposure to a Wi-Fi router and a mobile phone radiation simulator. As for the Wi-Fi router, it operated through the connection with a laptop located 5 meters away. The power of the router was 1 W and the SAR (absorption

rate) was 0.13 W / kg at 14 centimeters distance (place of exposure). Remember that SAR is an indicator of the extent to which our body absorbs that radiation. In the United States the legal limit is 2.0 W / kg, while in the European Union it is 1.6. Therefore, the bacteria were exposed to a level of absorption rate significantly lower than that stipulated as legally harmful.

As for the mobile phone, a 900 MHz GSM simulator was used, although in this case the authors did not indicate the emission power density or the SAR.

Samples of the bacteria were collected at 4 different

times of exposure: 3, 6, 9, and 12 hours, to compare their analysis with the control group (not exposed). This comparison is determined by the size of the zone of inhibition (its diameter), that is, the area around an antibiotic disk in which bacterial growth does not occur. In this way, the bacteria will be more resistant the less halo of inhibition present, since this makes the growth zone larger.

Results and implications

In the case of the E coli bacteria, it presented a pattern of response to the exposure time by which the The antimicrobial stay was significantly different than the control sample for the

4 time periods considered. Of the 48 comparisons made using the non-parametric Mann-Whitney U test (6 antibiotics x 4 time lapses x 2 types of exposure), only 8 were not significant.

Furthermore, the pattern of dose response was not linear, but apparently hormonal, where the maximum resistance was obtained for exposure doses between 6 and 9 hours.

However, in the case of Listeria bacteria, the results were not so clear, and only a clear effect was observed for the antibiotic doxycyclina.

Furthermore, the growth rate of both bacteria was higher

in the samples exposed to radiation compared to the control.

In this way, this research provides new evidence on the effects of electromagnetic fields on health, in this case through the increase in antimicrobial resistance, which represents one of the greatest challenges in current medicine, given the apparent increase of the resistance of some bacteria to a large portion of all known antibiotics. The authors postulate as a mechanism of action in cells the alteration of the sensitivity of cell membranes and ion exchange channels.

Limitations / Comments

The authors do not report data on exposure to the mobile phone simulator. This is a very relevant limitation because we do not know the intensity of the exposure, only the frequency. Although the frequency of the wave is proportional to the energy and is the one that produces the biological effect, the intensity tells us the speed or the level at which that change can occur, that is, it is a way of quantifying the effect for those levels. of energy. It is strange that in a magazine called "Dose-Response", the authors are not required to clearly specify the 900 MHz exposure dose, as they do

with the 2.4 GHz Wi-Fi
router.
Another important limitation
is the one related to the
statistical analysis since
they do not use a
correction of the
significance threshold due
to the multiple tests
carried out. Although this
fact, as we have commented
in other articles, is the
subject of debate in the
disciplines of epidemiology
and statistics, the results
could have been reported
with a correction of the
significance threshold
(smaller / more demanding
than 0.05), and compare
them with those already
specified.
Finally, I believe that this
research could have

provided more relevant results for this field if the authors had focused on a single antibiotic, and had replicated the experiment with that same antibiotic themselves. In this way, the endpoints would have been reduced, and a more forceful answer would have been given at the scientific level.

In any case, the indications that this research shows are again worrisome for human health and that threat posed by being continuously exposed to artificial electromagnetic fields, which although they are not ionizing, have negative biological effects, as hundreds and hundreds of investigations have been

showing in recent years.
From Martin Pall PhD,
Professor Emeritus of
Biochemistry and Basic
Medical Sciences,
Washington State
University.
Access my 90 page, seven
chapter document on EMF
effects, how they occur in
the body and corruption of
international science:
http://peaceinspace.blogs.com
/files/5g-emf-hazards-dr-
martin-l.-pall-eu-emf2018-
6-11us3.pdf
Chapter 7 of the book:
5G: Great health risk for the
EU, USA! USA And
international! Convincing
evidence of eight different
types of great harm caused
by exposure to
electromagnetic fields

(EMF) and the mechanism that causes them.

Chapter 7: The Big Risks of 5G: What We Know and What We Don't Know (See the book for references).

We have already discussed two questions that are essential to understanding 5G. One is that pulsed EMFs are, in most cases, much more biologically active than non-pulsed EMFs (often called continuous waves). And that EMFs work by putting forces on the voltage sensor of VGCCs, voltage-dependent calcium channels (VGCCs), opening these calcium channels and allowing excess calcium ions to flow into the cell. The voltage sensor is extremely sensitive to these electrical forces, so safety guidelines allow us to be exposed to EMFs that are something like 7.2 million times higher. The reason the industry has decided to go to the extremely high frequencies of 5G is that, with those extremely high frequencies, it is possible to transport much more information through much more pulsation than it is possible to transport at lower frequencies even in the microwave range. Therefore, we can be sure that 5G will involve much more pulsation than the EMFs to which we are currently exposed. It follows that any 5G biological safety test must use very fast pulsations, including very short-term spikes, which must be present in genuine 5G. There is an additional process that is planned to be used in 5G: phased arrays (https://en.wikipedia.org/wiki/Phased_array). Here, multiple antenna elements act together to produce highly pulsed fields that are designed for 5G, to produce greater penetration. 5G will involve particularly powerful keystrokes to be used, which can therefore be particularly dangerous.

The only data we have, to my knowledge, about 5G millimeter wave frequencies use unpulsed EMF in the 5G millimeter frequency range, not genuine 5G. Such millimeter waves have been shown to produce a number of subsequent effects of VGCC activation. A millimeter wave study showed that it activated both the VGCCs as well as the voltage-activated potassium channels, suggesting that it worked via the voltage sensor, just like other EMFs. Any of this data tells us next to nothing about how biologically active very highly pulsed genuine 5G will be.

I am assuming from your statements, that both Mr Ryan and Dr Vinciūnas are ready to launch 10 million 5G antennas to affect every person in the EU with 5G radiation without even a single genuine 5G biological safety test. . In the United States, the FCC, the Federal Communications Commission, has taken a much worse position. The FCC is not only willing to allow such completely untested exposures, but has also been aggressively lobbying to promote the installation of 5G antennas, so the antennas are already being installed in parts of the US. USA In a world where shocking behavior has become less and less shocking, I consider the views and actions of the EU and the US. USA they are shocking. The situation in the United States is massive madness. I would have hoped that Europeans, who consider themselves much more thoughtful than Americans, would have been actually more thoughtful.

Why does 5G need such a high number of antennas? This is because 5G radiation is absorbed much more as it enters various materials. The approach is to use many more antennas with one found every few houses, so that 5G can sufficiently penetrate local walls. Such absorption generally involves interaction with electrically charged groups, so such a high absorption is likely to involve placing forces on electrically charged groups. Because such forces are the way EMFs activate VGCCs, it seems highly likely, therefore, that 5G radiation is particularly active in activating VGCCs.

In summary, then, 5G is predicted to be particularly dangerous for each of the four different reasons:

The extraordinarily high numbers of antennas that are planned.

Very high power outputs to be used to ensure penetration.

Extraordinarily high pulsation levels.

4. The apparent high-level interactions of the 5G frequency in charged groups presumably including the charged groups of the voltage sensor.

The communications industry argues that 5G radiation will be absorbed mainly outside 1 or 2 mm from the body, so they claim that we don't have to worry about the effects. There is some truth to that, but there are also some caveats that make any conclusions drawn from that much more suspicious. In any case, these 5G surface effects will have an especially strong impact on organisms with much higher surface / volume ratios. Consequently, I predict that many organisms will be much more affected than we are. This includes insects and other arthropods, birds, and small mammals and amphibians. It includes plants that include even large trees, because the trees have leaves and reproductive organs that are very exposed. I predict that there will be major ecological disasters as a consequence of 5G.

This will include major conflagrations because EMF exposures make plants much more flammable.

But let's get back to humans. The industry has also claimed that more conventional microwave frequency EMFs have a limited effect on the outside of 1 cm from the body. We know this is not true, however, because of the profound effects on the human brain, heart, and hormonal systems. Perhaps the two most important studies demonstrating profound effects within the body are the studies by Professor Hässig and his colleagues in Switzerland on cataract formation in newborn calves. These two studies clearly show that when pregnant cows are grazing near At mobile phone base stations (also called cell phone towers), hatchlings are born with a very high incidence of cataracts. From these findings it follows that even though developing fetuses are very deep in the mother's body and must be highly protected from EMF exposures, they are not as well protected. And because EMF security guidelines in Switzerland are 100 times stricter than security guidelines in most of the rest of Europe, in the US. In the US, Canada, and most of the rest of the world, more general safety guidelines allow for exposure and penetration of effects. Industry claims that microwave frequency EMFs only act on the body's outer centimeter are clearly false.

How can conventional microwave frequency EMFs and 5G radiation act deep within the body? You can correctly observe that the electrical effects of EMFs activate the voltage sensor and that direct electrical forces are rapidly attenuated in the body. So how can we get deep effects? I think the answer is that the magnetic parts of electromagnetic fields have been known for decades to penetrate much deeper than electrical parts. Magnetic fields exert forces on electrically charged moving groups dissolved in the aqueous phases of the body, and small individual movements of charged groups can regenerate electric fields that are essentially identical to the electric fields of the original electromagnetic fields, carrying the same frequency and the same pulsation. pattern, although with less intensity. An example of this is given in

Lu and Ueno's study. Because the voltage sensor is so incredibly sensitive to electrical forces, and part of the reason is the high level of amplification of the electric field through the plasma membrane, we have an almost perfect way of producing EMF effects deep within our bodies. .

I am very concerned that 5G may produce effects like those we already see produced from low frequency EMF, but they are much more serious. I am also concerned that we will also see answers that are qualitatively different. Let me give you three possible examples of the latter type and a quantitative example. Each

of the four types of
blindness has side effects
of VGCC activation as
causal factors: cataracts,
detached retinas, glaucoma,
and macular degeneration.
Aqueous and vitreous
humors in the eye can be an
ideal environment for the
regeneration of electrical
fields within the eye.
Therefore, we can have a
gigantic epidemic of each of
the four types of blindness.
Another concern centers on
kidney dysfunction, which in
Chapter 5 was affected by
EMFs. The kidneys have a
lot of fluid, both blood and
what will become urine,
which can allow efficient
regeneration of electric
fields. Such regeneration
can be expected to affect

both glomerular filtration and reabsorption, both essential for kidney function.

Does this mean that 5G will produce very large increases in kidney failure? The only way to find out is to run genuine 5G radiation biological safety tests. Let me give you a third example. Fetuses and very young babies have much more water in their bodies than adults. Therefore, they can be a special risk for 5G impacts, due to large increases in the regeneration of electric fields. Here one can think of all kinds of possibilities. Let me suggest two. We may have a gigantic epidemic (sorry to use that

word again) of miscarriage
due to the teratogenic
effect.
Another possibility is that
instead of autism being a
birth at 38, as horrible as
it is, it could be one in two,
or even most births. I don't
know if this will happen, but
these are the types of risks
we are taking and there are
many others one can think
of. Putting in tens of
millions of 5G antennas
without a single biological
security test must be the
most stupid idea anyone has
ever had in the history of
the world.

UNIVERSAL DECLARATION
ON BIOETHICS AND
HUMAN RIGHTS
We highlight 3 of the articles.
Article 6 - Consent

1. All preventive, diagnostic
   and therapeutic medical
   intervention must only be
   carried out with the free
   and informed consent of
   the person concerned,
   based on the appropriate
   information. Where
   appropriate, consent should
   be express and the person
   concerned may revoke it at
   any time and for any
   reason, without this
   entailing any disadvantage
   or harm to him.

2. Scientific research should
   only be carried out with the

free, express and informed consent of the person concerned. The information should be appropriate, be provided in an understandable way and include the modalities for the revocation of consent. The interested person may revoke their consent at any time and for any reason, without this entailing any disadvantage or harm for them. Exceptions to this principle should be made only in accordance with the ethical and legal standards approved by the States, in a manner consistent with the principles and provisions set forth in this Declaration, particularly Article 27, and with international law relating to human rights.

3. In the cases corresponding to investigations carried out in a group of people or a community, the agreement of the legal representatives of the group or the community in question may also be requested. The collective agreement of a community or the consent of a community leader or other authority should in no way replace the informed consent of a person.

Article 27 - Limitations to the application of the principles

If limitations are to be imposed on the application of the principles set forth in this Declaration, it should be done by law, in particular the laws related to public safety to investigate, discover and prosecute crimes, protect public health and safeguard the rights and freedoms of others. Said law must be compatible with international human rights law.

Article 28 - Subject to interpretation: acts that go against human rights, fundamental freedoms and human dignity

Nothing in this Declaration may be interpreted as conferring on any State, group or individual any right to undertake activities or carry out acts that go against human rights, fundamental freedoms and human dignity.

HOW TO PROTECT YOURSELF FROM RADIATION, PRANYONES

Pranyons are the energy of the life force made up of photons, phonons, orgone energy and the amount of oxygen necessary for your body to assimilate. All of this is directed from the primary source of energy or the fohat.

You can create devices by intention and set the features you want to run.

Say mentally or out loud:

FOHAT PRANYONES GOLD RODS OF RA

And let the energy flow.

The rods of Ra incorporate the ancient geometric equation of the "Golden Section" or "Golden Mean". This sacred geometric relationship seems to have a beneficial effect on living organisms, which is not surprising given the fact that all growth in nature seems to follow this amazing and beautiful pattern of regeneration. The resulting number, 1.6180339 ... is incorporated into the Rods of Ra.

With this enhancement you can activate any object like orgonite but more powerful and effective in time and healing.

The most powerful results give the impression of being achieved by using the sticks of Ra for ten or fifteen minutes in a standing position, with the left foot forward, bare feet in contact with the ground, looking at the sun both at sunrise and sunset. The positive effect seems to be amplified when the body is properly hydrated by drinking plenty of water. Additionally, the benefits seem to increase by adding a small amount of Himalayan salt to drinking water, which appears to increase the body's electrical conductivity.

Say mentally or out loud:

PRANYONES DNA

And let the energy flow.

Here you activate the energy of the pranyonEs in your DNA, to heal, repair, channel, meditate, you activate your body as an antenna of light force energy.

Say mentally or out loud:
PRANYONS IRIDIUM
    MONOATOMIC
MONOATOMIC RHODIUM
    PRANYONS
MONATOMIC GERMANIUM
    PRANYONS
And let the energy flow.
This balances the strands of
    your DNA to give and
    receive energy from the
    light force. It also has an
    anti-aging effect and
    weight loss if necessary.
    Smooths the progress of
    the energy conversion-
    transformation in your
    bodies.
Say mentally or out loud
EMPOWERMENT TO THE
    PYRAMID CHAMBER OF
    PRANYONS
And let the energy flow.
Easily amplifies and

concentrates the life force
of energy. You can imagine
being inside an etheric
pyramid or anyone else for
regeneration as long as you
want. You can have a
pyramid item and energize
it with this empowerment.
You are empowered to use the
image that appears in this
text.
You can laminate it and use it
as a device with the
previous powers.
You can elixir with these
powers, like flower therapy
and more, just set the
intention with the energies
you want to put in.
You can load the elements
fire, water, earth, wind and
ether with these
properties. Pranyones have
amazing and wonderful

properties.
Say mentally or out loud:
EMPOWERMENT TO
  ELEMENTS OF PRANYONS
And let the energy flow.
Say mentally or aloud:
PRANYONS DNA INTRONS
  ZERO POINT-RADIONS
And let the energy flow.
With this power you can
  protect your DNA,
  biological and ethereal.
Say mentally or out loud:
PRANYONS RAY
  MITOCHONDRIAL ULTRA
  MAGENTA
This ensures the balance of
  energy in your cells with
  adequate EMF, biological
  and spiritual.
Our spiritual and gravitational
  center is Alcyone.
So we depend on the
  electromagnetic balance

To be in tune,
Say mentally or out loud:
Galactic Center of Gravity
     DNA-RNA BALANCE.
Say mentally or out loud
GRAVITATIONAL
     PRANYONS RAY
PRANYONS ACTIVATE
     SEROTONIN
This activates negative ions in
     your biological DNA
     structure and stimulates
     serotonin.
Say mentally or out loud:
PRANYONS CRYSTAL
     PHOTONIC-FONONIC
     MULTIDIMENSIONAL
This activates the harmonic
     electromagnetic fields with
     your biological structure
     aligning the frequencies of
     the earth and the cellular
     iron.

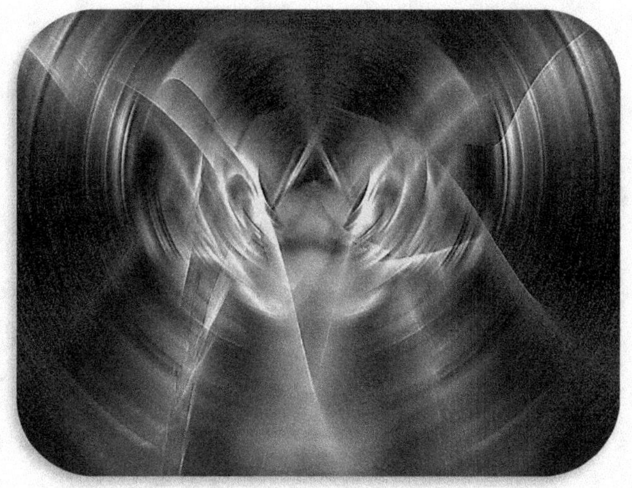

Disclaimer:

For legal reasons.

This report has been written
to provide information on
the damages of mobile or
cellular technology. If
medical attention is needed,
a competent professional
should be sought. The
purpose is to inform. The
author has no responsibility
if any person or entity
alleges damages caused
directly or indirectly
derived from the content
of this book.